CHRONIC SINUSITIS DIET FOR NOVICES

Discover Key Foods, Recipes, And Lifestyle Strategies To Conquer Chronic Sinus Issues And Enjoy Lasting Relief

DR. JACE ZAYDEN

Table of Contents

DISCLAIMER

The information provided in the book is intended for general informational purposes only. The content of this book should not be considered a substitute for professional medical advice, diagnosis, or treatment.

Readers are advised to consult with a qualified healthcare professional for medical advice tailored to their individual circumstances.

The author has made every effort to ensure that the information in this book is accurate and up-to-date at the time of publication. However, medical knowledge is constantly evolving, and new research may emerge that could impact the information presented. The author disclaims any responsibility for any adverse effects or consequences resulting from the use of the information provided in this book.

References or mentions of individuals, products, websites, organizations, or other names within this book are for informational purposes only and do not constitute an endorsement. The author has no affiliations with, and makes no endorsements of, any third-party entities mentioned. Readers are encouraged to conduct their own research and exercise their judgment when considering any external resources or recommendations.

The author and the publisher shall have neither liability nor responsibility to any person or entity with respect to any loss, damage, or injury caused or alleged to be caused directly or indirectly by the information contained in this book. Any reliance on the information within this book is at the reader's own risk.

By reading this book, the reader acknowledges and agrees to the terms of this disclaimer. If the reader does not agree with these terms, they should not use the information provided in this book.

ABOUT THIS BOOK

This book entitled "Chronic Sinusitis Diet" provides an all-encompassing resource for those who are enduring the difficulties associated with chronic sinusitis. By conducting a methodical examination of multiple aspects, this book offers indispensable knowledge regarding the treatment of this condition. The introductory segment provides an overview of chronic sinusitis and emphasizes the importance of adhering to a specialized diet as a means of managing the condition. Comprehending the intricacies of chronic sinusitis is critical for formulating an efficacious approach; this book skillfully explores this facet, furnishing readers with indispensable insights.

A central theme explored in this book pertains to the significance of diet in the management of chronic sinusitis. Acknowledging the significant influence that dietary decisions can exert on the health of the sinuses, this book provides an exhaustive account of the specific foods that ought to be incorporated and omitted from a diet for chronic sinusitis. An additional section is devoted to the significance of hydration in sinus health, underscoring the critical connection between sufficient water consumption and the mitigation of symptoms associated with the sinuses.

Furthermore, this book explores the domain of a specialized anti-inflammatory diet for chronic sinusitis, illuminating the possible advantages that may arise from the integration of anti-inflammatory food items. An extensive examination is also given to the importance of vitamins, minerals, herbal remedies, and supplements in promoting sinus health, providing readers with a holistic approach to managing their condition.

In addition to dietary considerations, this book explores modifications to one's lifestyle that may promote respiratory health. By incorporating a segment devoted to meal preparation for individuals with chronic sinusitis, the text assists its audience in applying pragmatic dietary approaches. An illustrative chronic sinusitis diet plan augments the practical utility of this book, furnishing readers with a concrete manual to assist them in navigating dietary modifications.

Elucidating prevalent fallacies and misunderstandings regarding chronic sinusitis enhances this book's clarity, thereby enabling readers to arrive at well-informed judgments. In conclusion, this book emphasizes the value of obtaining personalized guidance through consultation with healthcare professionals, in recognition of the collaborative nature of healthcare.

The "Chronic Sinusitis Diet" is an indispensable resource that integrates scientific knowledge with practical guidance to enable individuals to take an active role in managing their chronic sinusitis through dietary and lifestyle modifications.

CHAPTER ONE

Introduction

Chronic sinusitis is an inflammation of the sinuses that, despite medical treatment, persists for at least 12 weeks. A variety of symptoms may ensue, encompassing nasal congestion, facial discomfort, and respiratory distress. Although medical interventions such as nasal mists and antibiotics are frequently prescribed to treat chronic sinusitis, the importance of diet in this regard is becoming increasingly apparent. A nutrient-dense and harmonious diet can be of paramount importance in mitigating symptoms and averting reoccurrences. This article aims to provide an in-depth analysis of chronic sinusitis and emphasize the significance of incorporating a particular dietary regimen as a means of effectively managing this condition.

Comprehending Prolonged Sinusitis

Chronic sinusitis occurs when the cavities around the nasal passages, known as sinuses, become inflamed and distended for an extended period.

Numerous factors, including infections, sensitivities, and anatomical abnormalities like nasal polyps, can induce this inflammation. Chronic sinusitis is distinguished from acute sinusitis, which generally has a lesser duration, by its persistent character.

The symptoms of chronic sinusitis can be debilitating, impacting an individual's quality of life. Nasal congestion, facial pain or pressure, nasal breathing difficulties, and a diminished perception of scent or taste are typical symptoms. A persistent sensation of mucus trickling down the back of the pharynx (postnasal drip), fatigue, and cough are also common symptoms.

Managing chronic sinusitis often entails a multifaceted approach that may include medications, nasal irrigation, and, increasingly, dietary modifications. Although diet may not be a panacea, it can contribute to overall respiratory health and work in conjunction with other treatments.

The Significance Of Diet In Chronic Sinusitis Management

The influence of diet on chronic sinusitis management is substantial, owing to its effects on the immune system, inflammation, and general well-being. Specific food items may either promote or inhibit inflammation, thereby impacting the frequency and intensity of symptoms associated with sinusitis.

A diet low in inflammation may prove advantageous in the management of chronic sinusitis, as inflammation is a major contributing factor to this condition. Antioxidant-rich foods, including fruits and vegetables, have the potential to mitigate inflammation and bolster the immune system. Conversely, an excessive intake of processed foods, refined sugars, and saturated fats may exacerbate symptoms of sinusitis and contribute to inflammation.

In addition, it is imperative to maintain a healthy weight, as surplus weight has the potential to worsen respiratory problems and promote inflammation. A higher risk of developing chronic sinusitis is associated with obesity; therefore, weight loss via a balanced diet and consistent exercise can improve symptom management.

Additionally, hydration is a crucial component of dietary management for chronic sinusitis. Adequate hydration facilitates the thinning of mucus, thereby enhancing its drainage from the sinuses. Additionally, sufficient hydration aids the body's capacity to combat infections that could potentially contribute to sinusitis by promoting overall immune function.

Incorporating Foods Into A Diet For Chronic Sinusitis

Those who suffer from chronic sinusitis may find it advantageous to incorporate anti-inflammatory and immune-boosting nutrients into their diet. Consider incorporating the following essential ingredients into a diet for chronic sinusitis:

1. Fruits and Vegetables: Fruits and vegetables, being abundant in antioxidants, vitamins, and minerals, support the immune system and reduce

inflammation. Excellent options include berries, citrus fruits, asparagus, and leafy vegetables.

2. Flaxseeds, walnuts, fatty fish (salmon, mackerel, and trout), and flaxseeds are rich in omega-3 fatty acids, which possess anti-inflammatory characteristics.

3. Spices: Meals may include turmeric and ginger, which are recognized for their anti-inflammatory properties. These seasonings are suitable for both culinary use and tea infusions.

4. Lean Protein: Choose sources of lean protein, such as lentils, legumes, poultry and fish, among others. Protein is vital for immune function and tissue repair.

5. Probiotic-rich foods, including sauerkraut, yogurt, and kefir, can help maintain a healthy balance of intestinal flora. There exists a correlation between a robust immune system and a positive intestinal microbiome.

6. Opt for whole grains over refined cereals, such as quinoa, brown rice, and oats. Whole cereals furnish vital nutrients and dietary fiber, thereby promoting holistic well-being.

7. Maintaining adequate hydration throughout the day is crucial for promoting sinus drainage and maintaining thin mucus. Additionally, herbal broths and beverages can aid in hydration.

In summary, although diet in isolation may not offer a panacea for chronic sinusitis, the implementation of a nutritious and anti-inflammatory regimen can substantially aid in symptom management and the prevention of relapses. To ensure a comprehensive approach to managing chronic sinusitis and modify dietary recommendations to individual requirements, it is imperative to seek guidance from a registered dietitian or a healthcare professional. Through the process of making informed dietary decisions, individuals can exercise agency in safeguarding their respiratory health and general well-being.

Foods To Avoid

Chronic sinusitis, which is distinguished by inflammation of the sinus cavities that persists for a duration exceeding 12 weeks, has the potential to profoundly affect an individual's quality of life. Although medical remedies are indispensable, maintaining sinus health and managing symptoms can be significantly aided by a healthy diet. Specific foods have the potential to aggravate sinusitis symptoms and inflammation. An exhaustive list of foods to exclude from a diet for chronic sinusitis is provided below.

1. Dairy Products: Sinus congestion is frequently induced by dairy products. Mucus can become viscous when milk and other dairy products are consumed, preventing the sinuses from draining correctly. Reducing or eliminating dairy from the diet may alleviate obstruction and improve sinus drainage in individuals prone to sinus problems.

2. Refined sugar-rich foods have the potential to compromise immune function and induce inflammation. This includes sweetened beverages,

chocolates, and sugary treats. Insomnia symptoms may be exacerbated by chronic inflammation, which can be exacerbated by high blood sugar levels. For the health of the sinuses, substituting natural sweeteners or limiting sugar consumption may be beneficial.

3. Processed foods frequently comprise artificial ingredients, preservatives, and additives, all of which have the potential to induce inflammation. Due to the sodium content of processed foods, water retention may develop, which can exacerbate respiratory obstruction. Chronic sinusitis patients would benefit from consuming an unprocessed, whole-food-centered diet.

4. Gluten intolerance may be observed in certain individuals who have chronic sinusitis; gluten is a protein that is present in wheat, barley, and rye. An inflammation-causing symptom of gluten intolerance may also contribute to respiratory problems. Individuals who are experiencing chronic sinusitis symptoms may benefit from

investigating the possibility of adopting a gluten-free diet.

5. Spicy foods may elicit varying degrees of alleviation for individuals with sinus obstruction; however, some may encounter an exacerbation of symptoms in affected individuals. Chronic sinusitis patients may experience nasal passage irritation and inflammation exacerbation when consuming spicy foods. Keeping track of one's tolerance to piquant foods is vital for symptom management.

6. Alcohol: Dehydration of the body, including the sinus tissues, can result in impaired sinus drainage and denser mucus. Further, specific alcoholic beverages, such as beer and red wine, may contain histamines, which in susceptible individuals may induce symptoms of sinusitis. Alcohol consumption should be avoided or limited for individuals with chronic sinusitis.

7. Caffeine: Caffeine, which is present in certain beverages, coffee, and tea, can cause dehydration.

It is critical for individuals suffering from chronic sinusitis to ensure sufficient hydration to facilitate mucous reduction and enhance sinus functionality. Although a moderate amount of caffeine is generally regarded as permissible, it is unwise to consume it in excess.

8. Fatty and seared foods have the potential to induce inflammation in various bodily organs, including the respiratory passages. In addition to promoting sinus drainage and contributing to excessive mucus production, these foods may also do so. It is advantageous to utilize healthful culinary techniques, such as grilling or baking, and to consume omega-3 fatty acids from sources like fish. Potential benefits of eliminating or reducing the consumption of these foods in the diet for individuals with chronic sinusitis include symptom relief, inflammation reduction, and improved sinus health as a whole. Before making substantial dietary adjustments, it is vital to consult with a registered dietitian or a healthcare professional.

CHAPTER TWO

The Importance Of Hydration For Sinus Health

Adequate hydration is critical for the maintenance of overall health, and it is especially important for those who suffer from chronic sinusitis. To capture and eradicate irritants, the sinuses generate mucus. However, dehydration causes the mucus to thicken, which obstructs drainage and raises the risk of sinus congestion and infections. A comprehensive comprehension of the significance of hydration in sinus health is imperative for the effective management of chronic sinusitis.

1. Hydration functions as a natural decongestant, aiding in the maintenance of thin mucous that is more readily expelled from the sinuses. Water facilitates the alleviation of sinus congestion by acting as a natural decongestant. Sufficient hydration throughout the day maintains mucus thinness, which promotes efficient drainage and

decreases the probability of experiencing symptoms associated with sinusitis.

2. Preventing Sinus Infections: Dehydrated Individuals are more susceptible to infections, including sinusitis, which can compromise the immune system. Sufficient hydration enhances the body's ability to combat pathogens, thereby decreasing the likelihood of developing sinus infections. Sufficient consumption of water bolsters the body's innate defense mechanisms.

3. Nasal and Sinus Irrigation: External hydration in the form of nasal and sinus irrigation can be advantageous in conjunction with internal hydration. By moistening the nasal passages, saline solutions facilitate normal function and alleviate irritation. To maintain healthy sinuses, a neti pot or saline nasal rinse may prove to be effective mechanisms.

4. Continual Fluid Consumption: Although water serves as the principal hydration source, medicinal infusions, and clear broths may also

contribute to the overall fluid intake. Nevertheless, it is critical to exercise caution when consuming caffeinated and alcoholic beverages, given their potential diuretic properties that may result in heightened dehydration.

5. Tailored Hydration Requirements: The optimal daily quantity of water consumed differs between individuals. Age, weight, level of physical activity, and climate are all variables that affect hydration requirements. Although it is advisable to consume a minimum of eight 8-ounce containers of water daily, individual circumstances may dictate the need for adjustments.

6. The ability to identify indicators of dehydration is vitally important for individuals suffering from chronic sinusitis. Possible symptoms consist of increased thirst, parched mouth, vertigo, and dark urine. By monitoring hydration status and modifying fluid intake accordingly, complications associated with dehydration can be avoided.

7. Maintaining consistent hydration is a critical component in promoting the health of the sinuses. Consistently consuming water, particularly in arid or desiccated environments, can assist in preserving ideal moisture levels within the alveoli. Establishing a recurring schedule and, if required, integrating reminders can aid in accomplishing daily hydration objectives.

Adequate hydration is a straightforward yet effective method for managing chronic sinusitis. Sufficient fluid consumption can facilitate the production of thin mucous, avert sinus infections, and contribute to the overall well-being of the sinuses.

Implementing hydration practices into one's daily routine represents a proactive strategy for effectively managing symptoms of chronic sinusitis and enhancing overall health.

A Diet Low In Inflammation To Treat Chronic Sinusitis

Chronic sinusitis is frequently accompanied by inflammation; therefore, incorporating an anti-inflammatory diet into your regimen may prove to be an advantageous strategy in symptom management and the enhancement of overall sinus health. By emphasizing nutrients that reduce inflammation in the body, an anti-inflammatory diet may alleviate the symptoms of sinusitis. The benefits and fundamentals of an anti-inflammatory diet for chronic sinusitis are examined in this article.

1. Highlighting Fruits and Vegetables: Anti-inflammatory phytochemicals and antioxidants are abundant in vibrant fruits and vegetables. A varied selection of fruits and vegetables can aid in the reduction of inflammation and the mitigation of oxidative stress. Cruciferous vegetables, verdant greens, and berries are especially beneficial.

2. Omega-3 oily Acids: Flaxseeds, hazelnuts, and oily fish (salmon, mackerel, and sardines) are rich in omega-3 fatty acids, which have anti-inflammatory properties. By incorporating these omega-3 sources into the diet, sinusitis symptoms may be alleviated through modulation of the inflammatory response.

3. Opting for whole grains rather than refined grains offers the advantage of greater fiber content and a more diverse range of nutrients. A diet rich in whole grains, including quinoa, brown rice, and oats, is anti-inflammatory and nutritionally balanced. Additionally, fiber improves digestive health, which is associated with enhanced immune function.

4. Lean Proteins: Inflammation can be reduced by consuming lean protein sources, such as poultry, fish, legumes, and tofu. Fat and processed meats have the potential to induce inflammation; therefore, it is prudent to limit one's intake of these foods. Protein plays a critical role in immune function and tissue repair, thereby

bolstering the body's capacity to regulate sinusitis.

5. Herbs and Spices: Without relying on excessive amounts of sodium or sugar, numerous herbs and spices impart flavor to food and possess anti-inflammatory properties. Spices such as cinnamon, ginger, garlic, and turmeric have the potential to alleviate inflammation. By integrating these ingredients into recipes, one can augment the dietary benefits against inflammation.

6. Probiotics: Fermented foods containing probiotics, such as yogurt, kefir, and sauerkraut, supports a healthy balance of intestinal flora. A balanced microbiome in the intestine is associated with decreased inflammation and enhanced immune function. Consumption of foods abundant in probiotics is beneficial to overall health and may alleviate sinusitis symptoms.

7. Adequate hydration is a critical component to consider when following an anti-inflammatory

diet. Water aids in the drainage of waste products and facilitates the flushing of pollutants from the body. Additionally, hydration contributes to the maintenance of mucus's thin consistency, which facilitates sinus drainage.

8. Limiting Trigger Foods: It is equally critical to restrict or abstain from pro-inflammatory foods as it is to prioritize anti-inflammatory foods. This encompasses the consumption of refined carbohydrates, processed foods, and an inordinate amount of saturated and trans fats. By restricting the consumption of these trigger foods, one can enhance the efficacy of their anti-inflammatory regimen.

9. An individualized approach is necessary when designing an anti-inflammatory diet, as the response of each person to particular foods may differ, thus tailoring the diet to individual sensitivities and preferences. By keeping a food journal and observing the body's reactions to various foods, triggers can be identified and the diet can be adjusted accordingly.

10. It is recommended that individuals with chronic health conditions, such as sinusitis, consult with a registered dietitian or a healthcare professional before implementing substantial dietary modifications. They possess the ability to offer customized guidance, taking into account specific health requirements and possible drug interactions.

In summary, the implementation of an anti-inflammatory diet for chronic sinusitis necessitates the conscientious selection of foodstuffs, emphasizing whole, nutrient-rich foods that possess anti-inflammatory attributes. Although dietary interventions may not provide a definitive remedy for chronic sinusitis, they can be beneficial in symptom management and the promotion of sinus health as a whole. By incorporating these dietary principles into a comprehensive treatment regimen in conjunction with medical interventions, it is possible that a more holistic approach to managing chronic sinusitis could be achieved.

CHAPTER THREE

Minerals And Vitamins For Sinus Health

Chronic sinusitis, which is distinguished by ongoing inflammation of the sinuses, has the potential to vastly affect the quality of life of an affected individual. Sinus health can also be improved through the consumption of a balanced diet that is abundant in specific vitamins and minerals, in addition to the critical role that medical treatments play. These nutrients are of utmost importance in facilitating immune system function, mitigating inflammation, and fostering holistic health.

1. Vitamin C is essential for sustaining the health of mucous membranes, including those in the sinuses, due to its immune-boosting properties. Enhancing the body's resistance to infections, this vitamin may assist in the mitigation of sinusitis symptoms. Bell peppers, citrus fruits, and blueberries are all rich in vitamin C.

2. Vitamin A is an essential nutrient for the maintenance of respiratory system and mucous membrane health. As vitamin A is produced when the body converts beta-carotene, foods abundant in this compound (carrots, sweet potatoes, spinach, and sweet potatoes) may support respiratory health.

3. Vitamin E: Supporting the immune system and aiding in the fight against inflammation, vitamin E is an antioxidant. Spinach, almonds, and sunflower seeds are all excellent sources of vitamin E that may be incorporated into a diet designed to treat chronic sinusitis.

4. Zinc: Zinc is beneficial to respiratory health because it is essential for immune function and wound healing. Zinc-containing foods such as beef, lentils, and pumpkin seeds may help alleviate the severity and duration of sinusitis symptoms.

5. Magnesium, which is well-known for its anti-inflammatory properties, may assist in the relief

of chronic sinusitis symptoms. Magnesium-rich foods such as almonds, seeds, and verdant green vegetables can be integrated into a diet that is beneficial for the sinuses.

6. Quercetin, an inherent antioxidant with anti-inflammatory attributes, may prove advantageous in the management of symptoms associated with sinusitis. Onions, pears, and berries are examples of foods that are rich in quercetin.

7. Although probiotics do not qualify as vitamins or minerals, their contribution to respiratory health should not be disregarded. By promoting a healthy balance of intestinal flora, probiotics have the potential to impact the functioning of the immune system. Fermented foods, yogurt, and kefir are all rich in probiotics.

Although these vitamins and minerals may promote respiratory health, it is crucial to remember that they should be incorporated into a comprehensive diet. It is imperative to seek the advice of a healthcare professional before implementing substantial dietary modifications or supplementation.

Supplements And Natural Treatments

Herbal remedies and supplements, apart from vitamins and minerals, have garnered interest due to their potential efficacy in the management of symptoms associated with chronic sinusitis. Although scientific evidence may differ, the following may provide some individuals with relief:

1. Butterbur, scientifically known as Petasites hybridus, is a herb that possesses anti-inflammatory properties and potentially mitigates sinusitis symptoms. However, it is imperative to utilize a processed product to eliminate potentially hazardous compounds that may be present in unprocessed butterbur.

2. Bromelain, an enzyme that is present in pineapples, possesses anti-inflammatory characteristics. Bromelain supplements may aid in the reduction of nasal congestion and the

improvement of respiration in patients with chronic sinusitis, according to some studies.

3. The inhalation of vapor containing eucalyptus oil has the potential to alleviate nasal obstruction. The vapor produced by adding a few droplets of eucalyptus oil to heated water and inhaling it can assist in clearing the nasal passages.

4. Quercetin supplements are a viable option for individuals seeking to supplement their diets with the compound, which is also present in certain foods and may provide anti-inflammatory properties.

5. A neti pot, although not classified as an herbal remedy, can be utilized to eliminate mucus and allergens, thereby offering alleviation from sinus obstruction through the use of a saline solution. Sterilized or distilled water must be utilized to prevent complications.

Before adding any herbal supplements or remedies to your regimen, it is imperative that you seek the advice of a healthcare professional.

Certain substances may have contraindications or interact negatively with medications due to pre-existing health conditions.

Lifestyle Modifications To Promote Sinus Health

In addition to supplementation and dietary modifications, lifestyle adjustments can have a substantial impact on the management of chronic sinusitis. The following are some recommended practices:

1. Maintaining adequate hydration is critical to preserve the delicate consistency of nasal mucous. Eliminating the risk of sinus congestion by preventing mucous from becoming viscous and difficult to clear, adequate water consumption can aid in this regard.

2. Regular nasal irrigation with saline solution can facilitate the elimination of mucus and irritants, thereby enhancing the health of the sinuses. For this objective, saline nasal mists or neti pots may be utilized.

3. Humidification: By adding moisture to the air with a humidifier in your living space, you can prevent the nasal passages from drying out. This is especially advantageous in arid regions or throughout the winter, when the operation of indoor heating systems may result in arid air.

4. The importance of identifying and reducing allergen exposure cannot be overstated about respiratory health. This may encompass the utilization of air purifiers, consistent cleansing of living areas, and remediation of potential allergen sources such as pet dander and dust mites.

5. Consistent physical activity can elevate one's overall health, including the functionality of the immune system. Additionally, exercise improves circulation, which is advantageous for respiratory health.

6. The adverse effects of chronic stress on the immune system and inflammation necessitate stress management. The potential benefits of integrated stress management practices,

including yoga, meditation, and deep breathing exercises, on respiratory health should not be overlooked.

7. Preventing Irritatant Use: Tobacco smoke and various environmental contaminants have the potential to irritate the nasal passages, exacerbating symptoms of sinusitis. By preventing contact with these irritants, one can enhance the health of their sinuses.

It is critical to tailor these modifications to one's specific requirements and seek input from healthcare experts, including allergists or specialists in otolaryngitis, rhinitis, and pharyngitis, for individualized guidance.

CHAPTER FOUR

Preparing Meals To Manage Chronic Sinusitis

The development of a balanced dietary plan is of the utmost importance for those who are afflicted with chronic sinusitis. Key considerations for meal planning that promote respiratory health include the following:

1. To mitigate inflammation, incorporate anti-inflammatory foods into your diet. Fatty fish (salmon, mackerel) and flaxseeds are excellent sources of omega-3 fatty acids that can be found in abundance. Additionally, garlic, turmeric, and ginger are recognized for their anti-inflammatory properties.

2. Placing Emphasis on Fruits and Vegetables: An eating regimen abundant in fruits and vegetables furnishes vital antioxidants and vitamins. These can contribute to overall health and immune system support. Berry assortments, citrus fruits,

leafy vegetables, and bell peppers are all excellent examples of vibrant options.

3. Include foods high in lean protein, such as fish, chicken, tofu, and beans in your diet. Protein is vital for immune function and tissue repair.

4. Opt for whole cereals such as quinoa, brown rice, and whole wheat, which are rich in essential nutrients and fiber. The beneficial effects of fiber on digestive health have an indirect effect on respiratory health.

5. Consume probiotic-rich foods, such as fermented vegetables like sauerkraut, yogurt with live cultures, and kefir, to promote the health of the intestinal microbiome. Positive effects of a balanced intestinal microbiome on the immune system are possible.

6. Saturation is Critical: Sufficient water consumption is essential for nasal mucus to retain its thin consistency. Incorporate hydrating fruits, broths, and stews, which are high in water content, into your meal plan.

7. Restrict Trigger Foods: Certain foods may worsen the symptoms of sinusitis in some individuals. Dairy products, piquant foods, and processed foods are frequent triggers. It is advisable to monitor one's body's reaction to various foods and modify the meal plan accordingly.

8. Small, Regular Meals: Opt for substantial, time-consuming meals by incorporating smaller, more frequent meals into your daily routine. This may facilitate improved digestion and prevent excess.

9. Caffeine and alcohol have the potential to exacerbate sinus obstruction by causing dehydration. Both of these substances should be limited in intake. Adherence to moderation is crucial, and it is critical to supplement these beverages with sufficient water consumption.

10. It is advisable to seek personalized guidance by consulting with a registered dietitian or nutritionist. They possess the ability to assist in

the development of a customized meal plan that aligns with your requirements and dietary inclinations.

In summary, a comprehensive strategy for the management of chronic sinusitis encompasses a variety of lifestyle modifications, dietary supplements, individualized meal planning, and dietary decisions. Although certain individuals may find alleviation from these strategies, it is imperative to seek guidance from healthcare professionals to formulate a comprehensive and personalized management strategy. Consistent communication with healthcare providers is essential to ensure that adjustments to one's nutrition and lifestyle are in conjunction with medical treatments to achieve optimal sinus health.

A Strategy For Relief

Chronic sinusitis, which is distinguished by inflammation of the sinus passages that persists for a duration exceeding 12 weeks, has the potential to profoundly affect an individual's quality of life. Although medical interventions like nasal corticosteroids and antibiotics are frequently prescribed, the significance of diet in the management of chronic sinusitis is frequently disregarded.

In addition to medical treatments, a chronic sinusitis diet that is thoughtfully planned can help alleviate symptoms. This book aims to examine the significance of dietary decisions, present an illustrative diet plan for individuals with chronic sinusitis, debunk prevalent fallacies and misunderstandings, and underscore the criticality of seeking personalized guidance from healthcare professionals.

The Importance Of Diet In The Management Of Chronic Sinusitis

The management of chronic sinusitis is significantly influenced by diet, as specific nutrients have the potential to either intensify inflammation or aid in immune system support. By incorporating nutrients that stimulate the immune system and inhibit inflammation, sinus symptoms can be alleviated and overall health improved.

It is critical to prioritize foods that are abundant in nutrients and to avoid those that may aggravate or provoke symptoms of sinusitis.

Foods With Anti-Inflammatory Properties

1.Omega-3 fatty acids are anti-inflammatory substances that are present in walnuts, flaxseeds, and fatty fish (salmon, mackerel, and sardines). By incorporating these into one's diet, sinus inflammation may be alleviated.

2. Curcumin, the bioactive constituent of turmeric, has gained recognition for its anti-inflammatory properties. One should contemplate supplementing with turmeric or incorporating it into their meals in conjunction with a healthcare professional.

3. Blueberries, strawberries, and raspberries are rich in anti-inflammatory antioxidants. In

addition to being tasty, they are also advantageous for respiratory health.

4. Spinach, kale, and other verdant greens are abundant in anti-inflammatory antioxidants, vitamins, and minerals, all of which are beneficial to overall health.

Boosting The Immune System Foods

1. Citrus Fruits: Vitamin C, which is abundant in oranges, grapefruits, lemons, and limes, provides immune system support. Consistent intake can assist in the prevention and treatment of sinusitis.

2. Garlic and onions are aromatic vegetables that possess antimicrobial properties and potentially aid in the defense against infections. Incorporating these ingredients into one's diet may enhance overall immune health.

3. Yogurt and other fermented foods contain probiotics, which promote a healthy balance of intestinal flora. Optimal gastrointestinal health is associated with a more robust immune system.

4. Bell peppers, which are abundant in antioxidants and vitamin C, support immune system health. They lend vibrancy and adaptability to a variety of dishes.

CHAPTER FIVE

Dietary Plan For Chronic Sinusitis Example

While avoiding potential triggers, a dietary regimen for chronic sinusitis should include the aforementioned immune-boosting and anti-inflammatory foods. A sample diet plan for chronic sinusitis is provided below to assist with food selection:

Consuming Breakfast

• Option 1: Greek yogurt topped with a mixture of berries and a few flaxseeds.

• Oatmeal garnished with cut bananas and walnuts constitutes Option 2.

• Beverage: A sprinkle of lemon-infused green tea.

Convenience Snack

A small sprinkling of pistachios or other nuts, if desired.

• Beverage: Orange juice that has been freshly pressed.

• Grilled salmon salad featuring avocado, cherry tomatoes, and verdant greens constitutes Option 1.

Option 2: Quinoa concoction containing legumes and sautéed vegetables.

• Beverage: herbal tea or water infused with turmeric.

Savory Afternoon Meal

• Hummus with carrot and cucumber spears is an option.

• Beverage: A green smoothie comprised of pineapple, spinach, and ginger.

Consumed Dinner

Option 1: Chicken breast baked with quinoa and steamed broccoli.

2. Lentil soup accompanied by an assortment of leafy vegetables.

• The drink is ginger tea, served warm.

• A tiny bowl of assorted berries, if desired.

The beverage served is chamomile tea.

Typical Fallacies And Misconceptions

Similar to numerous health-related subjects, chronic sinusitis, and dietary management has been the source of numerous falsehoods and misunderstandings. To ensure that individuals receive accurate information and make well-informed decisions regarding their dietary choices, it is vital to debunk these misconceptions.

Myth 1: Dairy products invariably exacerbate sinusitis.

Although there are individuals who may develop an increased production of mucus in response to dairy, this is not a universal truth. A moderate amount of dairy, particularly low-fat varieties, does not worsen sinusitis in the majority of individuals.

Consistently monitoring one's reactions and seeking personalized guidance from a healthcare professional is imperative.

Myth 2: Sinusitis is exacerbated by spicy foods

Spicy foods, including those containing chile peppers, can, contrary to prevalent belief, aid in the relief of sinus congestion. Capsaicin, which is present in chiles, improves nasal drainage and thins mucus. On the contrary, those who have particular sensitivities should exercise caution when consuming piquant foods.

Contrary to Myth No. 3, allergies and sinusitis do not share identical dietary triggers.

Although certain dietary variables may cause allergies and sinusitis to overlap, these are two separate conditions that originate from different underlying factors. While this may be the case for allergy sufferers, it is unlikely to exert the same therapeutic effect on chronic sinusitis by avoiding specific foods. It is imperative to comprehend the precise stimuli associated with each condition to implement effective management strategies.

Myth 4: A healthy diet can be entirely replaced by supplements

Although supplements may offer relief from particular nutrient deficiencies, they ought not to be regarded as a substitute for a nutritionally balanced diet. The synergistic effects of the nutrients, fiber, and antioxidants found in whole foods promote overall health. It is important to use supplements in addition to a healthy diet, not instead of it.

Expert Guidance In The Healthcare Sector

Although chronic sinusitis diet plans may offer broad principles, there are considerable individual differences; therefore, it is critical to seek personalized guidance from healthcare professionals. A registered dietitian or a healthcare professional specializing in ear, nose, and throat (ENT) can evaluate your particular condition, take into account latent factors, and customize dietary suggestions to suit your specific requirements.

The Critical Role Of Expert Guidance

1. Individualized Evaluation: Healthcare practitioners can perform a comprehensive evaluation of your medical background, food allergies, and dietary inclinations to develop a strategy that is by your specific requirements.

2. Monitoring and Adjustments: Consistent consultations with healthcare practitioners facilitate the surveillance of your advancement and enable the implementation of dietary modifications by your body's reactions.

3. Trigger Identification: The assistance of healthcare professionals in identifying particular dietary triggers that could potentially worsen symptoms enables the implementation of more precise avoidance strategies.

4. Integration with Medical Treatment: To optimize the management of sinusitis as a whole,

a holistic approach entails the integration of dietary recommendations with medical treatments.

In summary, the incorporation of a balanced chronic sinusitis diet into one's regimen can significantly contribute to symptom management and the promotion of overall sinus health. By elucidating prevalent misconceptions and integrating foods that enhance the immune system and inhibit inflammation, individuals can empower themselves to make well-informed decisions that mitigate the adverse effects of chronic sinusitis. Nevertheless, it is critical to seek the advice of healthcare professionals to receive individualized guidance and guarantee that dietary interventions are by specific health requirements and medical factors.

Conclusion

In summary, the implementation of a meticulously customized dietary regimen can have a substantial influence on the control of chronic sinusitis. Although universally applicable, managing the condition by consuming anti-inflammatory foods, staying hydrated, and avoiding potential triggers can help mitigate symptoms and avert flare-ups.

By prioritizing a diet abundant in fruits, vegetables, and omega-3 fatty acids, one may potentially mitigate inflammation within the sinus passages, thereby facilitating improved drainage and ventilation. In addition, maintaining adequate hydration facilitates mucus thinning and promotes optimal mucus production, thereby simplifying the process of sinus clearance.

For some, it may be advantageous to reduce or eliminate from their diet processed or dairy products, which are known to aggravate sinusitis symptoms. Nevertheless, it is critical to seek guidance from a registered dietitian or a healthcare professional to develop an individualized dietary regimen that takes into account one's specific requirements and sensitivities.

Dietary modifications are ultimately incorporated into a holistic approach to chronic sinusitis management, in conjunction with other prescribed remedies by medical professionals. Chronic sinusitis relief requires lifestyle modifications, environmental adjustments, and appropriate medical interventions; all of these are critical components in this process. By integrating a nourishing and anti-inflammatory dietary regimen into a holistic therapeutic strategy, patients may experience an amelioration of symptoms and an enhancement of their overall quality of life.

THE END